The Liver Whisperer

A Step-By-Step Plan to Revitalize Your Liver, Detox Your Body, and Achieve Optimal Health

Dr. Keith Brady

Scan, to check out more of my publications.

Table of contents

Introduction

The liver is one of the most important organs in the body. It is responsible for over 500 vital functions, including detoxification, digestion, metabolism, and immunity. When the liver is healthy, it is able to perform these functions efficiently and effectively. However, when the liver is unhealthy, it can lead to a variety of health problems, including liver disease, fatigue, digestive problems, and weight gain.

The good news is that the liver is a very resilient organ and has the ability to heal itself. With the right support, you can revitalize your liver, detox your body, and achieve optimal health.

This book, The Liver Whisperer, will provide you with everything you need to know to heal your liver and optimize your health. You will learn about the liver's important functions, the signs and symptoms of liver disease, and the benefits of a healthy liver. You will also learn about the Liver Whisperer's 7-Day Liver Cleanse, the Liver Whisperer's Diet for Optimal Liver Health, and the Liver Whisperer's Guide to Liver Detoxing.

The Liver's Important Functions

The liver is involved in over 500 vital functions in the body, including:

- Detoxification: The liver removes toxins from the blood, such as alcohol, drugs, and environmental pollutants.
- Digestion: The liver produces bile, which helps to break down fats in the small intestine.
- Metabolism: The liver converts food into energy and stores nutrients such as glycogen, iron, and vitamins A, D, E, and K.
- Immunity: The liver produces antibodies and other immune cells that help to fight off infection.

The Signs and Symptoms of Liver Disease

Liver disease can be caused by a variety of factors, including viruses, alcohol abuse, fatty liver disease, and autoimmune diseases. The signs and symptoms of liver disease can vary depending on the cause, but some common symptoms include:

- Fatigue
- Jaundice (yellowing of the skin and eyes)
- Dark-colored urine
- Pale stools
- Abdominal pain and swelling
- Loss of appetite
- Nausea and vomiting
- Itchy skin
- Bruising easily
- Edema (fluid retention)

The Benefits of a Healthy Liver

A healthy liver is essential for overall health and well-being. The benefits of a healthy liver include:

- Increased energy levels
- Improved digestion
- Stronger immune system
- Better weight management
- Healthier skin
- Reduced risk of liver disease and other chronic diseases

The Liver Whisperer's 7-Day Liver Cleanse

The Liver Whisperer's 7-Day Liver Cleanse is a gentle and effective way to detoxify your liver and improve your overall health. The cleanse involves following a special diet and taking certain supplements to help your liver eliminate toxins and heal itself.

The Liver Whisperer's Diet for Optimal Liver Health

The Liver Whisperer's Diet for Optimal Liver Health is a whole-food, plant-based diet that is rich in nutrients and antioxidants. This diet is designed to support liver function and detoxification.

The Liver Whisperer's Guide to Liver Detoxing

In addition to the 7-Day Liver Cleanse, there are a number of other things you can do to detoxify your liver, such as:

- Eating a healthy diet
- Exercising regularly
- Avoiding alcohol and drugs
- Managing stress
- Getting enough sleep

The liver is a vital organ that plays a key role in overall health and well-being. By following the advice in this book, you can revitalize your liver, detox your body, and achieve optimal health.

How This Book Can Help You Achieve Optimal Liver Health

This book will provide you with the tools and knowledge you need to heal your liver and optimize your health. You will learn about the liver's important functions, the signs and symptoms of liver disease, and the benefits of a healthy liver. You will also learn about the Liver Whisperer's 7-Day Liver Cleanse, the Liver Whisperer's Diet for Optimal Liver Health, and the Liver Whisperer's Guide to Liver Detoxing.

This book is written in a clear and concise style and is easy to understand. It is also packed with practical advice and tips that you can implement

immediately to start improving your liver
health.

If you are serious about improving your liver
health, then this book is a must-read.

Chapter 1: The Liver Whisperer's 7-Day Liver Cleanse

What is a Liver Cleanse and Why is it Important?

A liver cleanse is a process of removing toxins from the liver. The liver is responsible for filtering toxins from the blood, but over time, these toxins can build up and damage the liver. A liver cleanse can help to remove these toxins and restore the liver to optimal health.

There are many different types of liver cleanses, but the Liver Whisperer's 7-Day Liver Cleanse is a gentle and effective way to detoxify the liver. This cleanse involves following a special diet and taking certain supplements to help the liver eliminate toxins and heal itself.

The Benefits of the Liver Whisperer's 7-Day Liver Cleanse

The Liver Whisperer's 7-Day Liver Cleanse offers a number of benefits, including:

- Improved liver function
- Reduced inflammation
- Increased energy levels
- Improved digestion
- Weight loss
- Clearer skin
- Reduced stress

What to Expect During the Cleanse

During the Liver Whisperer's 7-Day Liver Cleanse, you will follow a special diet that is designed to support liver function and detoxification. The diet includes plenty of fruits, vegetables, and whole grains, and it is low in processed foods, sugar, and unhealthy fats.

You will also take certain supplements during the cleanse to help the liver eliminate toxins and heal itself. These supplements include:

- **Milk thistle:** Milk thistle is a herb that has been shown to protect and repair the liver.
- **Dandelion root:** Dandelion root is a herb that helps to detoxify the liver and gallbladder.
- **Turmeric:** Turmeric is a spice that has anti-inflammatory and antioxidant properties.
- **Ginger:** Ginger is a herb that helps to improve digestion and reduce inflammation.

Step-By-Step Instructions for the Cleanse

Here are the step-by-step instructions for the Liver Whisperer's 7-Day Liver Cleanse:

Day 1:

- Eat a light breakfast of fruit and yogurt.

- At lunch, have a salad with grilled chicken or fish.
- For dinner, have steamed vegetables with brown rice.
- Take 2 milk thistle capsules and 1 dandelion root capsule before bed.

Day 2:

- Start your day with a green smoothie made with spinach, kale, banana, and avocado.
- At lunch, have a lentil soup with whole-grain bread.
- For dinner, have quinoa with roasted vegetables.
- Take 2 milk thistle capsules and 1 dandelion root capsule before bed.

Day 3:

- Eat a bowl of oatmeal with berries and nuts for breakfast.
- At lunch, have a turkey sandwich on whole-wheat bread with a side salad.
- For dinner, have salmon with roasted vegetables.

- Take 2 milk thistle capsules and 1 dandelion root capsule before bed.

Day 4:

- Start your day with a glass of warm lemon water.
- At lunch, have a bowl of vegetable soup with whole-grain crackers.
- For dinner, have grilled chicken breast with brown rice and steamed broccoli.
- Take 2 milk thistle capsules and 1 dandelion root capsule before bed.

Day 5:

- Eat a smoothie made with yogurt, berries, and protein powder for breakfast.
- At lunch, have a salad with grilled fish.
- For dinner, have lentil soup with whole-grain bread.
- Take 2 milk thistle capsules and 1 dandelion root capsule before bed.

Day 6:

- Start your day with a bowl of oatmeal with berries and nuts.
- At lunch, have a chicken salad sandwich on whole-wheat bread with a side salad.
- For dinner, have salmon with roasted vegetables.
- Take 2 milk thistle capsules and 1 dandelion root capsule before bed.

Day 7:

- Eat a light breakfast of fruit and yogurt.
- At lunch, have a salad with grilled chicken or fish.
- For dinner, have steamed vegetables with brown rice.
- Take 2 milk thistle capsules and 1 dandelion root capsule before bed.

Recipes for Liver-Cleansing Foods and Drinks

Here are some recipes for liver-cleansing foods and drinks:

Green Smoothie

Ingredients:

- 1 cup spinach
- 1 cup kale
- 1 banana
- 1/2 avocado
- 1 cup water

Instructions:

1. Combine all ingredients in a blender and blend until smooth.
2. Enjoy immediately.

Lentil Soup

- 1 onion, chopped
- 2 carrots, chopped
- 2 celery stalks, chopped
- 1 teaspoon garlic powder
- 1/2 teaspoon salt
- 1/4 teaspoon black pepper

Instructions:

1. Rinse the lentils in a fine-mesh strainer.

2. In a large pot, combine the lentils, vegetable broth, onion, carrots, celery, garlic powder, salt, and pepper.
3. Bring the soup to a boil, then reduce the heat to low and simmer for 20-30 minutes, or until the lentils are tender.
4. Serve hot.

Roasted Vegetables

Ingredients:

- 1 pound vegetables of your choice, such as broccoli, carrots, Brussels sprouts, sweet potatoes, or zucchini, cut into bite-sized pieces
- 1 tablespoon olive oil
- 1/2 teaspoon salt
- 1/4 teaspoon black pepper

Instructions:

1. Preheat the oven to 400 degrees F (200 degrees C).
2. Toss the vegetables with the olive oil, salt, and pepper.
3. Spread the vegetables in a single layer on a baking sheet.

4. Roast the vegetables for 20-30 minutes, or until they are tender and browned.
5. Serve immediately.

Salmon with Roasted Vegetables

Ingredients:

- 1 pound salmon fillet
- 1 tablespoon olive oil
- 1/2 teaspoon salt
- 1/4 teaspoon black pepper
- Roasted vegetables (see above)

Instructions:

1. Preheat the oven to 400 degrees F (200 degrees C).
2. Brush the salmon fillet with olive oil and season with salt and pepper.
3. Place the salmon fillet on a baking sheet and roast for 15-20 minutes, or until cooked through.
4. Serve the salmon with roasted vegetables.

Liver-Cleansing Drinks

Here are some recipes for liver-cleansing drinks:

Beetroot Juice

Ingredients:

- 1 beet, peeled and chopped
- 1 apple, peeled and chopped
- 1 carrot, peeled and chopped
- 1/2 inch ginger, peeled and chopped
- 1 cup water

Instructions:

1. Combine all ingredients in a juicer and juice until smooth.
2. Enjoy immediately.

Dandelion Tea

Ingredients:

- 1 teaspoon dried dandelion root
- 1 cup water

Instructions:

1. Add the dandelion root to a cup of hot water.
2. Steep for 10 minutes.
3. Strain and enjoy.

Turmeric Tonic

Ingredients:

- 1 teaspoon turmeric powder
- 1/2 teaspoon ground black pepper
- 1 cup hot milk of your choice

Instructions:

1. Combine the turmeric powder, black pepper, and milk in a mug.
2. Stir until well combined.
3. Enjoy immediately.

The Liver Whisperer's 7-Day Liver Cleanse is a gentle and effective way to detoxify the liver and improve overall health. By following the instructions in this chapter, you can complete the cleanse safely and successfully.

Here are some additional tips for completing the cleanse:

- Drink plenty of water throughout the day.
- Get enough sleep.
- Exercise regularly.
- Avoid alcohol and drugs.
- Manage stress.

If you have any questions or concerns about the cleanse, please consult with your doctor.

Chapter 2: The Liver Whisperer's Diet for Optimal Liver Health

The Importance of Diet for Liver Health

Diet is one of the most important factors for liver health. The liver is responsible for metabolizing the foods we eat, and the types and amounts of foods we eat can have a significant impact on liver function.

A healthy diet for the liver is one that is low in processed foods, sugar, and unhealthy fats, and high in fruits, vegetables, and whole grains. It is also important to limit alcohol intake and to avoid smoking.

Foods to Eat for Liver Health

Here are some of the best foods to eat for liver health:

- **Fruits:** Fruits are packed with vitamins, minerals, and antioxidants that are essential for liver health. Good choices include berries, apples, bananas, grapes, and citrus fruits.
- **Vegetables:** Vegetables are another important source of nutrients for the liver. Good choices include leafy greens, broccoli, cauliflower, Brussels sprouts, and beets.
- **Whole grains:** Whole grains are a good source of complex carbohydrates, fiber, and other essential nutrients that support liver health. Good choices include brown rice, quinoa, oats, and whole-wheat bread and pasta.
- **Lean protein:** Lean protein sources, such as chicken, fish, beans, and tofu, are essential for liver health. Protein helps to repair and rebuild liver tissue.
- **Healthy fats:** Healthy fats, such as those found in avocados, nuts, seeds, and olive oil, are important for liver function and overall health.

Foods to Avoid for Liver Health

Here are some foods to avoid for liver health:

- **Processed foods:** Processed foods are often high in unhealthy fats, sugar, and salt, and they can be low in nutrients. Processed foods can damage the liver and make it difficult for the liver to function properly.
- **Sugary drinks:** Sugary drinks, such as soda, juice, and sports drinks, are high in fructose, which can damage the liver. Fructose is converted to fat in the liver, and this can lead to fatty liver disease.
- **Unhealthy fats:** Unhealthy fats, such as saturated and trans fats, can damage the liver and lead to fatty liver disease. Unhealthy fats are found in fried foods, processed foods, and red meat.
- **Alcohol:** Alcohol is a toxin that can damage the liver. Heavy alcohol consumption can lead to alcoholic liver disease, which is a serious and potentially life-threatening condition.

Sample Meal Plans and Recipes for a Liver-Healthy Diet

Here are some sample meal plans and recipes for a liver-healthy diet:

Breakfast

- Oatmeal with berries and nuts
- Yogurt with fruit and granola
- Eggs with whole-wheat toast and avocado

Lunch

- Salad with grilled chicken or fish
- Lentil soup with whole-grain crackers
- Sandwich on whole-wheat bread with lean protein, vegetables, and healthy fats

Dinner

- Salmon with roasted vegetables
- Chicken stir-fry with brown rice
- Quinoa salad with black beans and vegetables

Recipes

Here are some recipes for liver-healthy meals and snacks:

Berry Smoothie

Ingredients:

- 1 cup berries (fresh or frozen)
- 1 banana
- 1 cup yogurt
- 1 cup milk of your choice

Instructions:

1. Combine all ingredients in a blender and blend until smooth.
2. Enjoy immediately.

Chicken Salad Sandwich

Ingredients:

- 2 slices whole-wheat bread
- 1/2 cup cooked chicken, shredded
- 1/4 cup mayonnaise
- 1 tablespoon Dijon mustard
- 1/4 cup chopped celery
- 1/4 cup chopped onion
- 1/4 cup chopped walnuts
- Salt and pepper to taste

Instructions:

1. Spread mayonnaise on one slice of bread.
2. Top with chicken, celery, onion, and walnuts.
3. Season with salt and pepper to taste.
4. Top with the other slice of bread.
5. Cut in half and enjoy.

Salmon with Roasted Vegetables

Ingredients:

- 1 pound salmon filet
- 1 tablespoon olive oil
- 1/2 teaspoon salt
- 1/4 teaspoon black pepper
- Roasted vegetables

Instructions:

1. Preheat the oven to 400 degrees F (200 degrees C).
2. Brush the salmon filet with olive oil and season with salt and pepper.
3. Place the salmon filet on a baking sheet and roast for 15-20 minutes, or until cooked through.
4. Serve the salmon with roasted vegetables.

Quinoa Salad with Black Beans and Vegetables

Ingredients:

- 1 cup quinoa, rinsed
- 2 cups water
- 1/2 cup black beans, rinsed and drained
- 1/2 cup corn kernels
- 1/2 cup diced red onion
- 1/4 cup chopped cilantro
- 1 tablespoon lime juice
- 1 tablespoon olive oil
- Salt and pepper to taste

Instructions:

1. Cook the quinoa according to package directions.
2. In a large bowl, combine the cooked quinoa, black beans, corn, onion, cilantro, lime juice, olive oil, salt, and pepper.
3. Mix well and enjoy.

The Liver Whisperer's Diet for Optimal Liver Health is a healthy and delicious way to support liver function and overall health. By following the tips in this chapter, you can create a liver-healthy diet that is right for you.

Here are some additional tips for following the Liver Whisperer's Diet for Optimal Liver Health:

- Eat plenty of fruits, vegetables, and whole grains.
- Choose lean protein sources, such as chicken, fish, beans, and tofu.
- Limit processed foods, sugary drinks, unhealthy fats, and alcohol.
- Drink plenty of water throughout the day.
- Get enough sleep.
- Exercise regularly.
- Manage stress.

If you have any questions or concerns about the Liver Whisperer's Diet for Optimal Liver Health, please consult with your doctor or a registered dietitian.

Chapter 3: The Liver Whisperer's Guide to Liver Detoxing

What is Liver Detoxing and Why is it Important?

Liver detoxing is the process of eliminating toxins from the liver. The liver is responsible for filtering toxins from the blood, but over time, these toxins can build up and damage the liver. Liver detoxing can help to remove these toxins and restore the liver to optimal health.

There are many different ways to detox the liver. Some common methods include:

- Diet: Eating a healthy diet is one of the best ways to detox the liver. A liver-healthy diet is low in processed foods, sugar, and unhealthy fats, and high in fruits, vegetables, and whole grains.
- Exercise: Exercise is another great way to detox the liver. Exercise helps to increase circulation and to stimulate the

lymphatic system, which helps to remove toxins from the body.

- Supplements: There are a number of supplements that can help to detox the liver. Some common supplements include milk thistle, dandelion root, and turmeric.
- Saunas: Saunas can also help to detox the liver by promoting sweating. Sweating helps to remove toxins from the body through the skin.

The Liver Whisperer's Guide to Liver Detoxing

The Liver Whisperer's Guide to Liver Detoxing is a comprehensive guide to detoxifying the liver. This guide includes information on all of the different liver detoxing methods, as well as a personalized liver detox plan.

Personalized Liver Detox Plan

The Liver Whisperer's Personalized Liver Detox Plan is a 7-day plan that is designed to help you detox your liver and improve your overall health. The plan includes:

- A liver-healthy diet
- A moderate exercise routine
- A list of recommended supplements
- A sauna schedule

Instructions for Following the Liver Whisperer's Personalized Liver Detox Plan

To follow the Liver Whisperer's Personalized Liver Detox Plan, simply follow the instructions below:

Diet

- Eat a liver-healthy diet that is low in processed foods, sugar, and unhealthy fats, and high in fruits, vegetables, and whole grains.
- Sample meal plans and recipes are provided in Chapter 2.

Exercise

- Exercise for at least 30 minutes most days of the week.
- Moderate-intensity exercise, such as brisk walking or swimming, is ideal.

Supplements

- Take the following supplements daily:
  - Milk thistle: 500 mg
  - Dandelion root: 500 mg
  - Turmeric: 500 mg

Sauna

- Use a sauna for 20-30 minutes 3-4 times per week.

Additional Tips

- Drink plenty of water throughout the day.
- Get enough sleep.
- Manage stress.

The Liver Whisperer's Guide to Liver Detoxing is a comprehensive guide to detoxifying the liver and improving overall health. By following the personalized liver detox plan, you can remove toxins from your liver and restore your liver to optimal health.

Here are some additional tips for liver detoxing:

- Avoid alcohol and drugs.
- Eat small, frequent meals throughout the day.
- Avoid eating late at night.
- Drink herbal teas, such as green tea and dandelion tea.
- Eat cruciferous vegetables, such as broccoli, cauliflower, and Brussels sprouts.
- Eat citrus fruits, such as oranges, lemons, and grapefruit.
- Eat beets and carrots.

If you have any questions or concerns about liver detoxing, please consult with your doctor.

Recipes for Liver Detox Drinks

Here are some recipes for liver detox drinks:

Dandelion Root Tea

Ingredients:

- 1 teaspoon dried dandelion root
- 1 cup water

Instructions:

1. Add the dandelion root to a cup of hot
   water.
2. Steep for 10 minutes.
3. Strain and enjoy.

Turmeric Tea

Ingredients:

- 1 teaspoon turmeric powder
- 1/2 teaspoon ground black pepper
- 1 cup hot milk of your choice

Instructions:

1. Combine the turmeric powder, black
   pepper, and milk in a mug.
2. Stir until well combined.
3. Enjoy immediately.

Beet Juice

Ingredients:

- 1 beet, peeled and chopped

- 1 apple, peeled and chopped
- 1 carrot, peeled and chopped
- 1/2 inch ginger, peeled and chopped
- 1 cup water

Instructions:

1. Combine all ingredients in a juicer and juice until smooth.
2. Enjoy immediately.

Following the Liver Whisperer's Guide to Liver Detoxing can help you to remove toxins from your liver and improve your overall health. By eating a healthy diet, exercising regularly, taking supplements, and using a sauna, you can detox your liver and restore it to optimal health.

Be sure to drink plenty of water throughout the day and to get enough sleep. You should also manage stress and avoid alcohol and drugs.

Eating small, frequent meals throughout the day, avoiding eating late at night, and drinking herbal teas such as green tea and dandelion tea can also help to detox your liver.

Eating cruciferous vegetables such as broccoli, cauliflower, and Brussels sprouts, citrus fruits such as oranges, lemons, and grapefruit, and beets and carrots can also help to detox your liver.

If you have any questions or concerns about liver detoxing, please consult with your doctor.

Chapter 4: The Liver Whisperer's Guide to Stress Management for Liver Health

The Link Between Stress and Liver Health

Stress is a normal part of life, but too much stress can have a negative impact on your liver health. When you're stressed, your body releases stress hormones, such as cortisol. Cortisol can damage liver cells and make it difficult for the liver to function properly.

Chronic stress can also lead to unhealthy behaviors, such as overeating, drinking alcohol, and smoking. These behaviors can further damage the liver and lead to liver disease.

The Best Stress Management Techniques for Liver Health

There are a number of stress management techniques that can help to protect your liver health. Some of the best techniques include:

- **Exercise:** Exercise is a great way to reduce stress and improve liver health. Aim for at least 30 minutes of moderate-intensity exercise most days of the week.
- **Relaxation techniques:** Relaxation techniques, such as deep breathing, meditation, and yoga, can help to reduce stress levels and improve liver function.
- **Time management:** Learning how to manage your time effectively can help to reduce stress and improve your overall well-being.
- **Social support:** Spending time with loved ones, talking to a therapist, or joining a support group can provide you with the social support you need to cope with stress.

Creating a Stress Management Plan for Liver Health

The first step to creating a stress management plan for liver health is to identify the sources of stress in your life. Once you know what's causing you stress, you can start to develop strategies for coping with it.

Here are some tips for creating a stress management plan for liver health:

- **Set realistic goals:** Don't try to do too much at once. Start by setting small, achievable goals.
- **Make time for relaxation:** Schedule time each day for relaxation activities, such as deep breathing, meditation, or yoga.
- **Learn to say no:** It's okay to say no to commitments that you don't have time for or that will add to your stress levels.
- **Delegate tasks:** If you have too much on your plate, delegate tasks to others.
- **Take breaks:** Take breaks throughout the day to relax and recharge.

- **Get enough sleep:** When you're well-rested, you're better able to cope with stress.
- **Eat a healthy diet:** Eating a healthy diet can help to improve your mood and reduce stress levels.
- **Exercise regularly:** Exercise is a great way to reduce stress and improve liver health.

Stress management is an important part of liver health. By following the tips in this chapter, you can create a stress management plan that works for you and helps to protect your liver health.

If you are feeling overwhelmed by stress, please talk to your doctor or a mental health professional. They can help you to develop a stress management plan and provide you with the support you need.

Here are some additional tips for stress management:

- **Avoid caffeine and alcohol:** Caffeine and alcohol can worsen anxiety and make it difficult to manage stress.

- **Spend time in nature:** Spending time in nature has been shown to reduce stress and improve mood.
- **Listen to music:** Listening to calming music can help to reduce stress and promote relaxation.
- **Get a massage:** Massage is a great way to reduce stress and improve muscle tension.

By following these tips, you can reduce stress and improve your overall health, including your liver health.

Chapter 5: The Liver Whisperer's Guide to Supplements for Liver Health

The Importance of Supplements for Liver Health

Supplements can play an important role in supporting liver health. A number of supplements have been shown to protect the liver from damage, improve liver function, and promote liver healing.

The Best Supplements for Liver Health

Some of the best supplements for liver health include:

- **Milk thistle:** Milk thistle is a herb that has been shown to protect and repair the liver. Milk thistle contains a compound called silymarin, which has antioxidant and anti-inflammatory properties.

- **Dandelion root:** Dandelion root is a herb that has been shown to detoxify the liver and gallbladder. Dandelion root also contains diuretic properties, which can help to flush out toxins from the body.
- **Turmeric:** Turmeric is a spice that has anti-inflammatory and antioxidant properties. Turmeric has been shown to protect the liver from damage and to improve liver function.
- **Ginger:** Ginger is a herb that has anti-inflammatory and antioxidant properties. Ginger has been shown to improve digestion and to reduce inflammation in the liver.

Other Supplements that May Benefit Liver Health

In addition to the supplements listed above, there are a number of other supplements that may benefit liver health, including:

- **NAC:** NAC (N-acetylcysteine) is an amino acid that has antioxidant and anti-inflammatory properties. NAC has been shown to protect the liver from damage and to improve liver function in people with liver disease.

- **Alpha-lipoic acid:** Alpha-lipoic acid is an antioxidant that has been shown to improve liver function and to reduce inflammation in the liver.
- **Choline:** Choline is an essential nutrient that helps the liver to metabolize fats. Choline deficiency can lead to fatty liver disease.
- **B vitamins:** B vitamins are important for liver function. B vitamins help the liver to metabolize fats, carbohydrates, and proteins.

How to Choose the Right Supplements for Liver Health

When choosing supplements for liver health, it is important to select high-quality products from reputable manufacturers. It is also important to talk to your doctor before taking any supplements, especially if you have any underlying health conditions or are taking any medications.

Dosage and Safety of Supplements for Liver Health

The dosage of supplements for liver health will vary depending on the individual. It is important to follow the dosage instructions on the product label or as directed by your doctor.

Supplements are generally safe when taken as directed. However, some supplements may interact with certain medications or cause side effects in some people. It is important to talk to your doctor before taking any supplements.

Supplements can play an important role in supporting liver health. A number of supplements have been shown to protect the liver from damage, improve liver function, and promote liver healing.

If you are considering taking supplements for liver health, it is important to talk to your doctor first. They can help you to choose the right supplements and to determine the appropriate dosage.

Here are some additional tips for using supplements for liver health:

- Take supplements with food to improve absorption.
- Avoid taking supplements with caffeine or alcohol, as these substances can interfere with absorption.
- Drink plenty of water throughout the day to help the body flush out toxins.
- Get regular blood tests to monitor your liver function.

By following these tips, you can safely and effectively use supplements to support your liver health.

Conclusion

The liver has a remarkable ability to regenerate. Even after significant damage, the liver can repair itself and restore its function.

The liver's regenerative ability is due to a process called hepatocyte proliferation. Hepatocytes are the main cells in the liver. When hepatocytes are damaged, they can divide to create new cells. This process of cell division allows the liver to repair itself and grow back to its original size.

The liver's regenerative ability is also due to a process called liver regeneration factor (LRF). LRF is a protein that is produced by the liver and other organs. LRF signals to hepatocytes to divide and repair the liver.

The liver's regenerative ability is important for overall health. A healthy liver is essential for digestion, metabolism, and detoxification. When the liver is damaged, it can lead to a number of health problems, including liver disease.

There are a number of factors that can affect the liver's regenerative ability. These factors include:

- **Age:** Younger people tend to have a better ability to regenerate their liver than older people.
- **Overall health:** People with good overall health tend to have a better ability to regenerate their liver than people with poor overall health.
- **Severity of liver damage:** The more severe the liver damage, the more difficult it is for the liver to regenerate.

There are a number of things that can be done to support the liver's regenerative ability. These include:

- **Eating a healthy diet:** A healthy diet provides the liver with the nutrients it needs to repair itself.
- **Getting regular exercise:** Exercise helps to improve liver function and promote liver regeneration.
- **Avoiding alcohol and drugs:** Alcohol and drugs can damage the liver and make

it more difficult for the liver to regenerate.

- **Getting enough sleep:** Sleep is essential for liver health and regeneration.
- **Managing stress:** Stress can damage the liver and make it more difficult for the liver to regenerate.

If you have liver disease, it is important to work with your doctor to develop a treatment plan that includes lifestyle changes and medications. With proper treatment, most people with liver disease can live long and healthy lives.